Healing Through Butter and Buttermilk

Healing Naturally with Milk Products

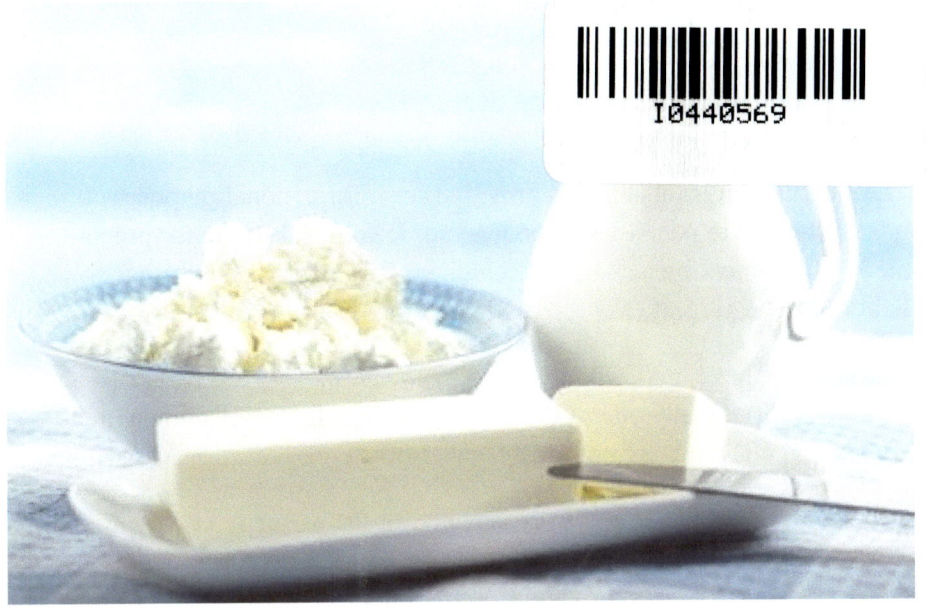

Dueep Jyot Singh

Healthy Living Series

Mendon Cottage Books

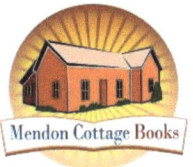

JD-Biz Publishing

Our books are available at

1. Amazon.com

2. Barnes and Noble

3. Itunes

4. Kobo

5. Smashwords

6. Google Play Books

Table of Contents

Introduction

There is a historical story about how man got to know about butter and buttermilk. Millenniums ago, when man was still a nomadic traveler, herding his sheep, goats, horses, and camels, along with him, when he traveled in search for a more suitable dwelling, the milk obtained from milking his domestic animals was stored in leather bags.

So as the story goes, one fine dawn two leather bags with lots of camels milk was stored on both sides of such a nomad's saddle, and the tribe moved off towards richer horizons and pastures. By the time the journey was done at dusk, and the leather bags were taken off, so that the thirsty traveler could drink up deep and gratefully, he found that there was some solid portion accumulated on top of the liquid.

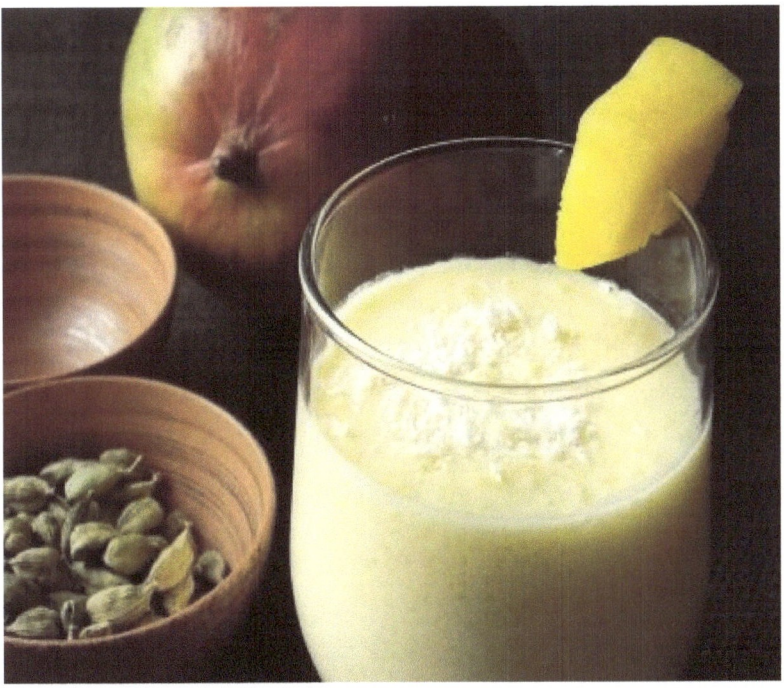

The loping motion of the camel, throughout the day had churned and agitated the milk in such a manner, that the milk had turned into buttermilk, and with lots of delicious solid butter floating on top of it.

Since then, mankind has blessed camels for adding another delicious, nourishing, healing food item to their daily meals.

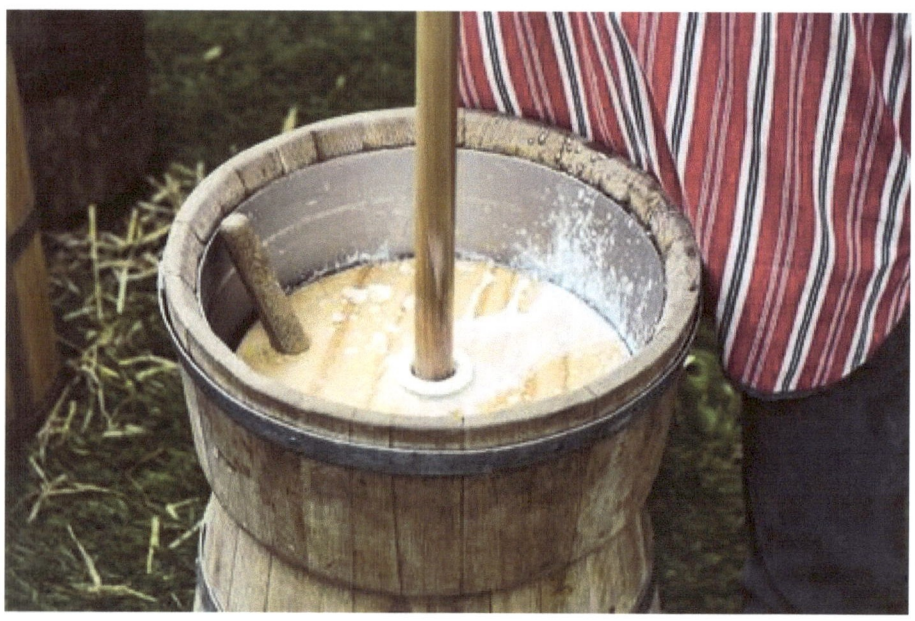

So this book is going to tell you all about how you can make fresh butter and buttermilk, as well as use it naturally and often, in order to heal yourself of a large number of ailments for which, otherwise, you would have taken the supposedly only other available option, of pills and other chemical-based drugs.

Buttermilk

In ancient times, it was believed that anybody who drank lots of buttermilk every day would never fall sick. Also, if buttermilk was used to cure diseases permanently, they would not reemerge again, if you stopped drinking buttermilk. In many ancient civilizations, it was considered to be the food of the gods, given to man, just as a gift because the gods supposedly were happy with mankind.

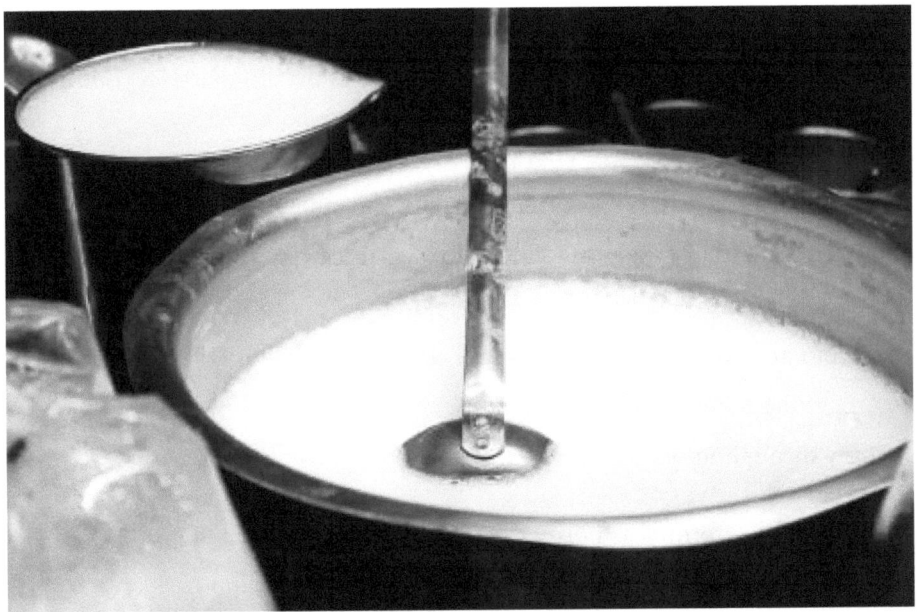

I was just looking through some ancient Indian medical treatises, written in Sanskrit, in which the praise of buttermilk was given in these words – if there was buttermilk available in Heaven, Lord Vishnu would not be dark in complexion! Also, the moon God would not have suffered from TB, the Fire

God would not have felt such a powerful burning sensation, and the king of the Gods would not have suffered from Piles.

Interesting how the gods suffered from ailments afflicting mankind, but could not be cured because there was no buttermilk around! Incidentally, I was more interested in the idea that buttermilk could make a person fair in complexion. This is something which has been proven down the ages and people of a dark complexion can lighten their skin tone, by applying buttermilk regularly on their face and hands, and drinking it in copious quantities.

Buttermilk is excellent for strengthening your immune system. It is also a good anti-toxic agent, getting rid of all the toxins accumulated in your body.

The best buttermilk is never made out of sour yogurt, if you are making it by churning yogurt, water, and cream together. In ancient times, buttermilk was drank with breakfast and with lunch in order to get the full benefit of its curative qualities. The best time for drinking buttermilk was at the end of a meal, or early in the morning. At night time you drank milk, three hours before going to sleep, and before you went to sleep, you drank water to keep healthy throughout your life.

In the West, buttermilk is normally made by churning day-old milk with water. Traditionally, it was done in a churn and it was supposed to be stylish having French Queens practicing to be dairy maids in their own home farms, in their palaces, churning butter while wearing satin and lace.

Nevertheless, buttermilk has been one of the most important food items, known to man, used to cure him of a large number of ailments. It is said that if a person is fed buttermilk since childhood, he is going to have a healthy youth and the gray-haired stage is going to come very late in life, no pun intended.

Making Butter and Buttermilk Out Of Cream

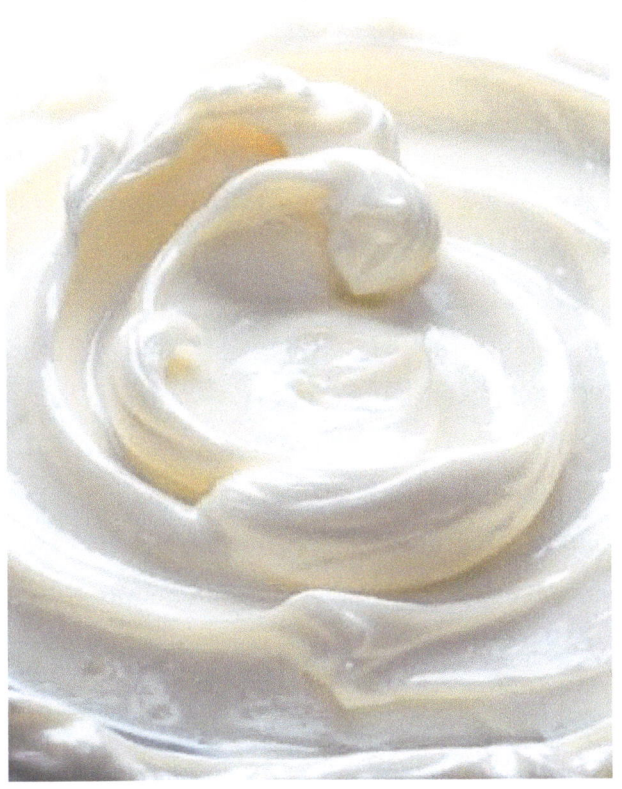

The top cream layer, on boiled milk is collected, and allowed to keep for a couple of days, so that the probiotic bacteria can flourish in them. So the day, when you want to make fresh butter, you take all this cream, and put it in the blender with some water. The water is going to separate, and you are going to have lumps of unsalted butter.

Can you make butter from fresh cream? Yes you can, but you are going to note the different quality of the butter made from "stale" cream, as compared to fresh cream butter. That is because fresh cream does not have many lactic acid bacteria in it, yet. But as it is, that cream is going to ferment and produce more and more lactic bacteria.

Also, if you make butter from cream with more lactic bacteria, it is going to increase the shelf life of the final product. That is because the bacteria do not allow any other bacteria to grow in their vicinity.

Buttermilk in Asia is the liquid, which is left over after the cream and the yogurt are churned with water.

Traditional Ancient Buttermilk Recipe

2 cups rich creamy yogurt
2 Equal amount of crushed ice or iced water
Two table spoons honey – if you want it sweet
Pepper and salt to taste
Half a teaspoonful of roasted roughly ground cumin seeds – if you want it salty

Since ancient times in the East, when there were no mixers and blenders around, all these items were placed in a huge churn and churned by hand until the mixture was frothy. The side product was of course fresh butter, which would then be scooped off and placed in clay containers.

This buttermilk was then topped off with a slice of cream or yogurt and served as an excellent digestive, with lunch in summer, or just drank whenever you feel thirsty, to prevent you from getting dehydrated in the hot summer sun.

Ailments treated through buttermilk

Diabetes Control

People suffering from diabetes can control this dread disease by drinking one glass of buttermilk, early in the morning before they eat or drink anything else. After 10 minutes, they need to drink a glass of fresh tomato juice. Try out this combination for three weeks, and you are going to find a visible change in your sugar levels.

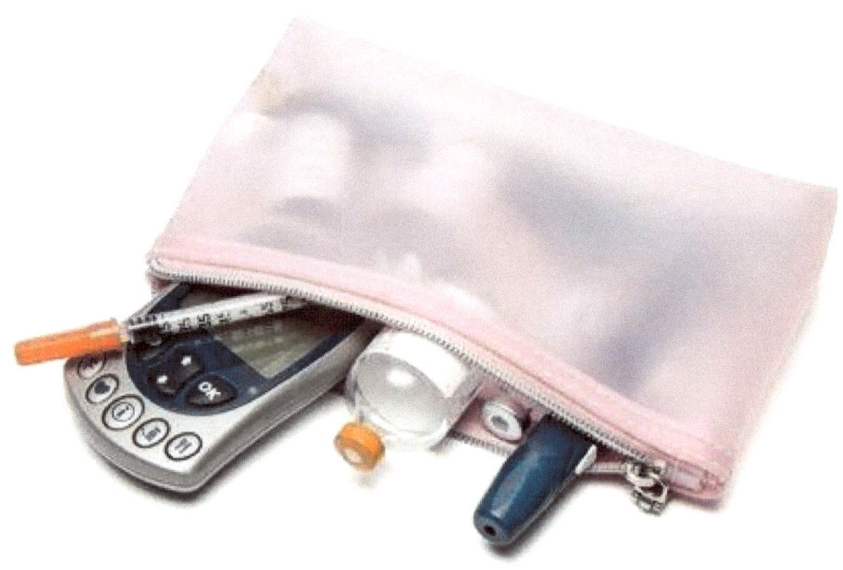

Piles

Take a glassful of buttermilk, and add rock salt to taste. Now add one tablespoonful of ground Bishops Weed spice. It is also known all over the world as "Ajowan". This mixture is a time-tested remedy to get rid of hemorrhoids and piles because the buttermilk cures the body from inside.

You can also add a little bit of roasted and ground cumin seeds to this mixture for better taste and a faster cure. Drink this every day for a week, to see an improvement. In fact, I can recommend drinking it twice a day, with breakfast and with lunch to detoxify your body and to help cure you faster.

Here are some spices which are going to help you cure piles – dry ginger - ground, green coriander, aniseed, and cumin seeds. Beneficial vegetables are the Indian gooseberry and Yams. These are starchy tubers, which are found extensively in the South Pacific, Asia, Africa, the Caribbean region, and in Latin America.

If you get yams easily, add them to your diet today, and you are never going to suffer from piles again. If the piles are bleeding, you will need to add rock salt and ground cumin seeds to the buttermilk and drink it – one glassful – four times a day until you are cured completely.

Flatulence

This is a delicious way in which you can get rid of flatulence forever. Just take one glass of buttermilk with a little bit of rock salt, half a spoonful of ground Bishops weed, at lunchtime. Drink this for about three weeks, and you are never going to suffer from flatulence or digestive problems again.

Diarrhea

People suffering from diarrhea just need to take two glasses of buttermilk, and add 1 tablespoon full of honey. Drink this, three times a day, empty bracket – that means six glasses of buttermilk and 3 tablespoons full of honey at four hour intervals – and it is going to cure the bacterial infection causing the diarrhea.

Or you can make a diarrhea remedy, ready for use, and bottled up, whenever a person suffers from an upset stomach.

Grind equal amounts of coriander seeds, aniseed, and cumin seeds after roasting them. Roasting fastens the essential oils in the seeds, and make them more powerful acting. Now add some rock salt to taste. Grind all four of these items into a very fine powder and put them in a glass bottle.

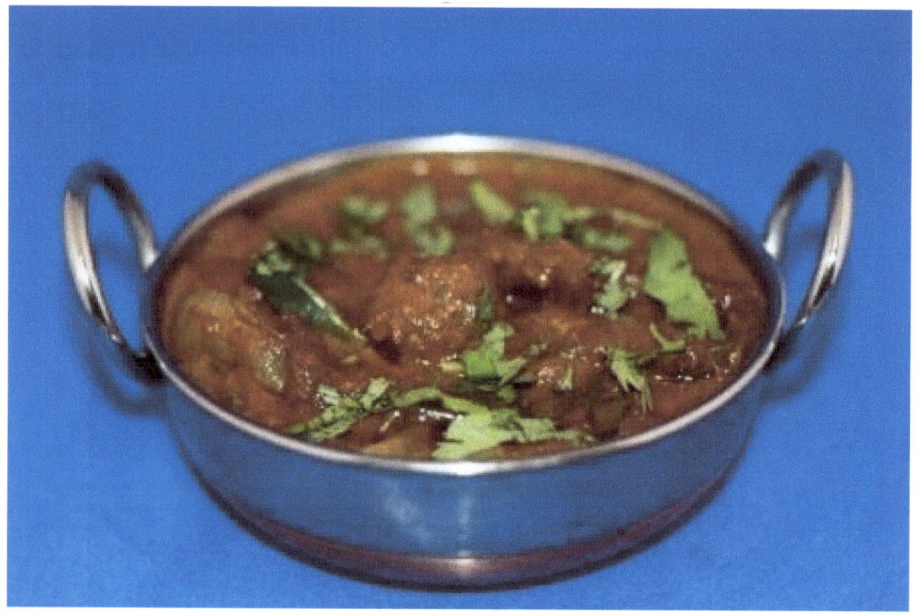

Too much rich and spicy food means your stomach can get upset, along with possible diarrhea.

Whenever somebody suffers from an upset stomach, just give him half a teaspoonful of this magic healing powder, in one glass of buttermilk. He will have to drink this, three times a day, and by the next day, he is going to be fit and fine. However, if the chronic case of diarrhea has been prolonged and the infection has been allowed to incubate for a number of days, he will need to take this treatment for three days. That gets rid of the infection as well as make sure that the body is not dehydrated due to essential mineral loss.

Chronic diarrhea – people suffering from chronic diarrhea can also take these powdered spices roasted in [clarified butter](#). Two pinches of Rock salt, half a teaspoonful of cumin seeds, and a touch of asafetida roasted, until they begin to give out their natural aroma. Powder them very finely, and make them into a mixture. Sprinkle half a teaspoonful of this mixture into a glass of buttermilk, and drink this four times a day.

Acidity

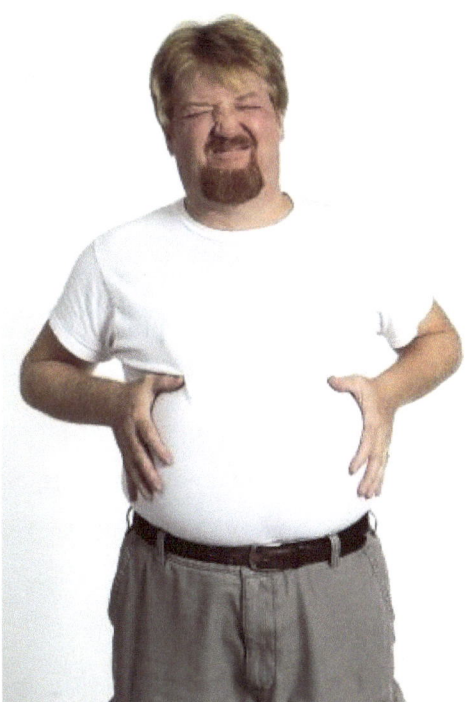

People suffering from acidity, especially, when they have been eating spicy food can cure, and also help prevented, by drinking one glass of buttermilk with 8 ground peppercorns of pepper and rock candy. According to taste. Drink this every two hours, five times a day. That means five glasses of buttermilk. This gets rid of the acidity. Also, you may wish to increase the consumption of milk, to help heal the ulcers caused in the intestinal passage, due to the acidity.

Swelling of the Stomach – Ascites

If you are suffering from ascites, which normally happens when there is an infection in your stomach region, stop eating spicy and rich food immediately. Now take 21 leaves of basil – neither more, nor less, and start chewing them. In between chewing, take sips of buttermilk. This is going to help cure all the infections in the stomach, causing ascites.

According to ancient medical treatises, these are the diseases, of mankind, which have been cured permanently through timeworn remedies, advocating the regular drinking of buttermilk.

High blood pressure, low blood pressure, gout, asthma, malaria, and urinary problems, including stones in the liver and in the urinary bladder. In fact, whenever I find myself suffering from any sort of stomach problem, including constipation or food not being digested just because I splurged on fatty stuff, I add a bit of roasted powdered cumin seeds, eight peppercorns, half a teaspoonful of dried mint, and two pinches of rock salt all powdered up to my glassful of buttermilk, and drink it down. Within 30 minutes, I find my system clearing up, wondrously.

People suffering from urinary problems, due to urinary infections can try this out. Add green coriander leaves to your glassful of buttermilk. If you are suffering from uric acid problems, these problems are going to be cured permanently by drinking buttermilk regularly. Also, people suffering from joint problems can be benefited immensely by drinking buttermilk.

Gout and Pain in the Back

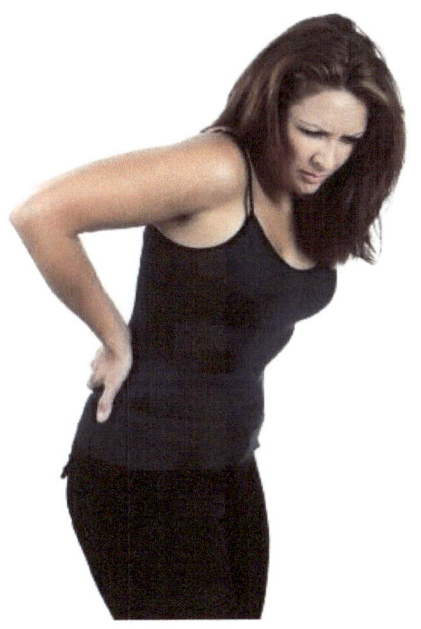

This was a remedy given to me by a friend, whose father suffered from gout, and she suffered from pain in the back and in the waist region. Incidentally, these remedies cured both of them! Take 10 peppercorns, and seven – eight cloves of garlic. Grind them well, and filter them in a muslin cloth. Pressing the cloth is going to get out garlic juice with peppercorns mixed in it. Mix the juice in a glass every day. This is going to cure your back problem and your pain in the waist region, permanently.

For the gout cure, she fed her father equal amounts of dried ginger powder, cumin seeds, black pepper, bishops weed, black and rock salt, all powdered up and mixed with a glassful of buttermilk. I would suggest a pinch of each and all of that is going to make half a teaspoonful! Drink this three times a day.

Gout is normally due to the presence of uric acid crystals in the body, and it is very painful. The buttermilk is going to get rid of the uric acid crystals, and cure you of gout. But you have to do this drinking three times a day, along with the healing spices cure, until you are completely healed. That is about the time it takes for the uric a city crystals to dissolve under the powerful onslaught of buttermilk.

Migraine

If you are suffering from a migraine problem, all you have to do is eat white rice for breakfast. This should be accompanied with buttermilk in which you have added a little bit of rock salt. This is going to cure your migraine, permanently.

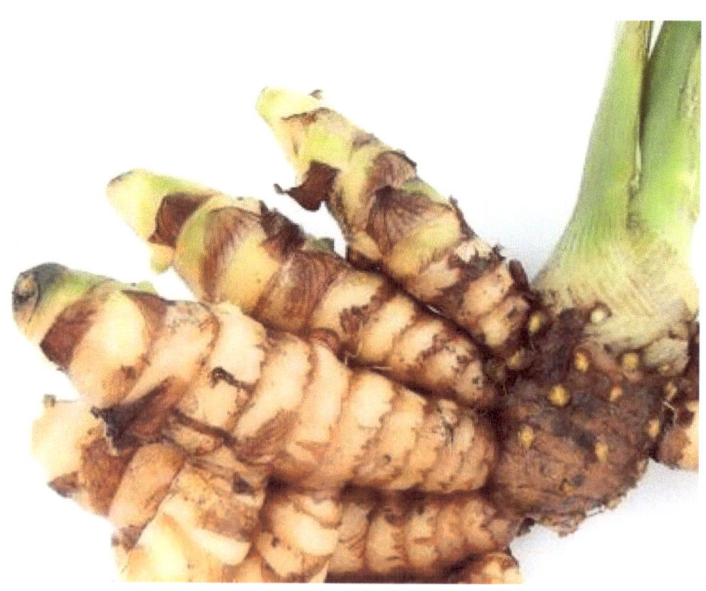

Let me give you one suggestion – make up a mixture of roasted bishops weed, rock salt, and pepper. Add this mixture to the buttermilk, whenever you drink it, and you are going to find a general increase of good health. If you want, you can also add a little bit of dried ginger to this mixture, especially when you are drinking it in the winter. The dried ginger is going to give you more warmth and boost up your immune system.

Urticaria

If you are suffering from this rash, which is normally made up of painful and itching weals – these normally occur, if you are allergic to some foods – you can cure this by soaking a piece of cotton in milk and dabbing it all over the affected area. Along with that, you are going to take 25 g of ground bishops weed and 25 g of molasses.

Mix them up well and divide them into two parts. In the morning, you are going to take one part of this, with fresh buttermilk and the other part is going to be eaten in the evening, with a glassful of water. Eat light food, porridge for choice or any other light food. This is going to cure the rash.

Cough and Cold

Buttermilk is excellent for a wet cough. Especially, when you are suffering from a chest infection and find that nasty phlegm being coughed up, whenever you have a coughing fit. You need to take instant measures so that the infection does not get chronic. Take a glassful of buttermilk, and add 1 tablespoon full of ground bishops weed to it. Drink this thrice a day, until you are cured of that nasty infection.

In fact, in ancient times, people suffering from chest problems including TB were given lots of buttermilk to drink, so that they could be cured naturally.

Buttermilk for Weight Loss

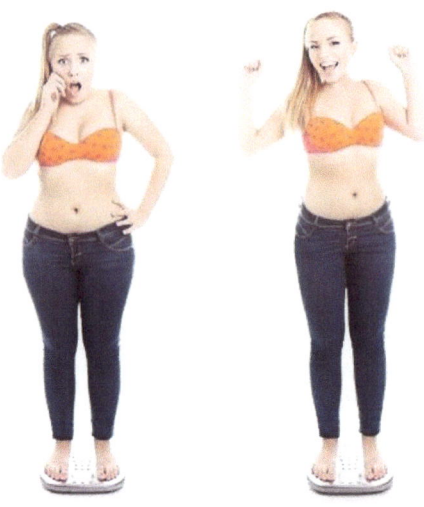

This is something which people who are always bothering about reducing weight are going to find very beneficial. Buttermilk is excellent for reducing weight ,drink one glass of buttermilk in which you have added 2 tablespoons full of honey, every morning first thing in the morning. You can then follow it up with one glass of lemon juice in warm water, with 1 tablespoon full of honey, after half an hour.

You may also want to "roast" the buttermilk on a hot griddle pan. This is done by heating up the griddle pan, and then when it is hot, throw a glassful of buttermilk on the heated surface. Switch off the heat immediately. Take this roasted buttermilk in a glass, and add rock salt to taste to it.

Use any of these remedies to reduce weight, whichever you find easier.

So now you are going to ask me, how much buttermilk do you need to drink in order to keep healthy. The answer is, there is absolutely no hard and fast rule, on how much buttermilk you can drink because after all, it is a healthy natural drink. In fact, children can drink up to half a liter of buttermilk and you can drink up to 1 L of buttermilk every day without it doing you any harm at all.

Butter

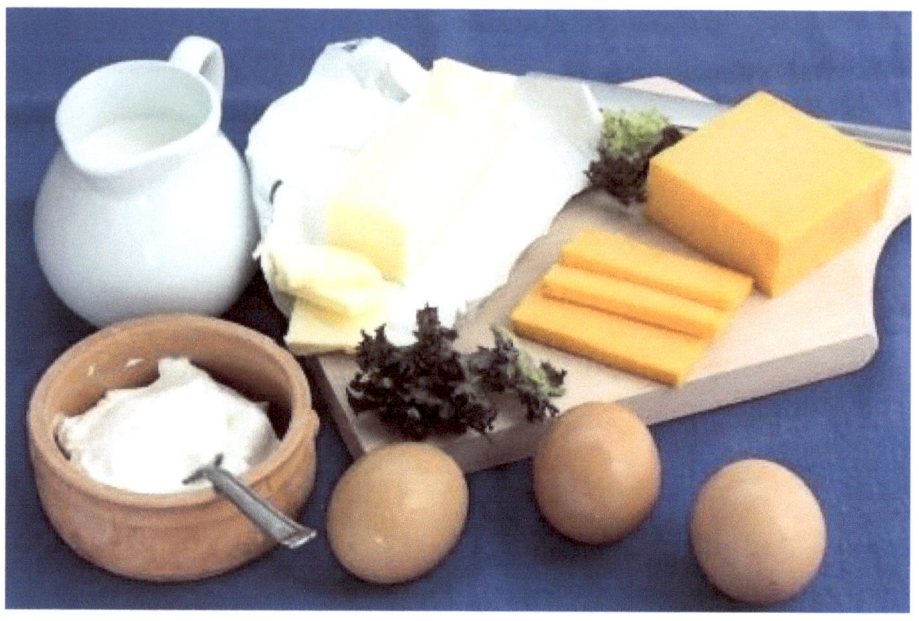

Homemade butter is of course best, because what you get in the market has a number of preservatives and chemical additives added to it, to help it last on the shelves for a longer period of time than what comes natural.

When I was young, I knew that I could scratch myself, moving about in the woods, with impunity, because when I came back, I was always scrubbed well with hot water to get rid of all the dust and grime and all my scratches and cuts treated with a mixture of homemade butter. Incidentally, none of them left scars. This was the ancient remedy and cure, to treat wounds, infections and cuts. If you lived, 2000 years ago and if clarified butter, which was an even more powerful concentrated form of butter was not available to heal you, your ancient wise grandmother would just dip into her churning bowl or churn, take out some butter, wash the wound with water, and then apply the butter all over it.

She would leave it un-bandaged to heal in the open air, if it was just a scratch. However, if the wound was deep, a piece of cotton cloth was taken, and a mixture of butter, honey and turmeric spread over the surface. That cotton cloth was then bound to the wound. Every morning, it was opened up to see the fresh tissue healing and the healthy healing mixture replaced on the wound, which was then bound up again.

So the next time you find yourself scratching yourself accidentally, do not reach out for any healing ointments which may perhaps have some Cortizone in it.

Here is one tip, which you are going to find useful, regarding Cortizone. This is excellent for skin diseases and ailments – doctors are going to recommend ointments with Cortizone and tar oil for fungal infections on the skin – but if you have an open cut or wound, never apply any ointment which has Cortizone in it. This aggravates the wound and it is never going to heal.

Measles and Chickenpox

If you are suffering from measles and chickenpox, naturally, you are going to find yourself itching a lot. Apply homemade butter on the itching area in order to moisturize it, and to prevent it from scarring. Let it be exposed to the air, because covering it with bandages is going to prevent the spots from drying up naturally.

If the patient is feeling feverish because of measles and chickenpox, you may want to take equal quantities of butter and rock candy. Take two spoons full of this mixture, first thing every morning until you are cured completely of fever.

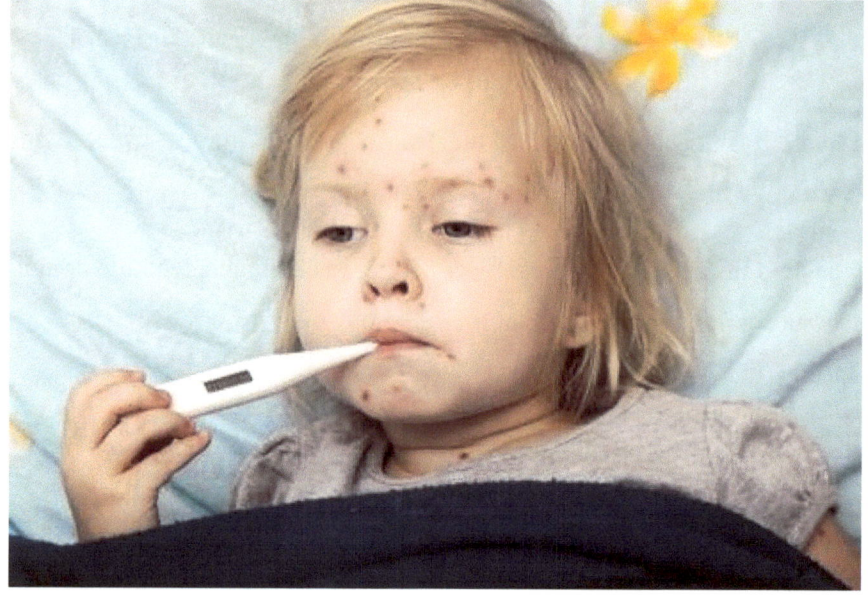

Traditional Clarified Butter – Desi Ghee

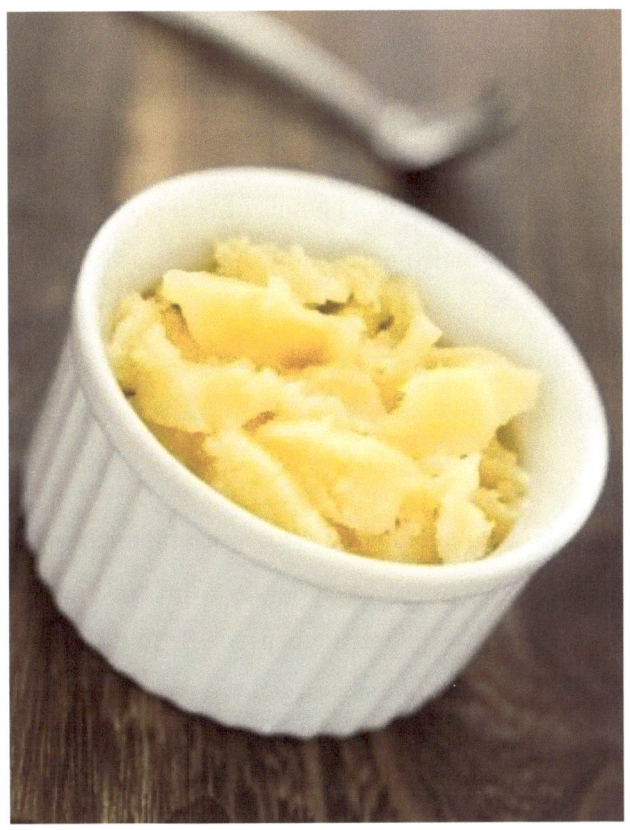

Desi ghee is clarified butter, which is extremely concentrated and a very powerful healing agent. It is normally used in the making up of herbal medicines, because it is made of pure creamy milk butter. It is also used in making beauty creams, potions, lotions, and other skin ointments.

It has a powerful aroma, and that is why only just a spoonful is added to fry meats. It is going to float on the surface of the meat dish, after it has been cooked, so you need to stir the gravy before serving. Also, the food is not going to taste greasy, even though it looks like it has been swimming in fat.

Desi ghee is the concentrated form of pure butter, which is heated to reduce the butter of all the impurities as well as moisture. This concentrated butter is normally used in Eastern cuisine, for searing meat, sautéing, and frying food, because desi ghee offers a higher burning point.

You make this at home by taking 2 pounds of best unsalted butter and melting it in a heavy bottomed pan. Allow the butter to liquefy on low heat for about 40 minutes. Maintain this simmering point, until all of the moisture in the butter has evaporated. The impurities are going to sink to the bottom of the pan. Remember to keep stirring the butter, so that it does not burn.

Pour off the clear butter and strain it through several thicknesses of muslin cloth. This butter is going to last for about a year, if it is placed in a cool and dry place. This butter is exorbitantly expensive. So in the East, people with easy access to plenty fresh milk make it right in their kitchens for crisp delicious frying results, and adding that taste of pure butter to all their dishes.

Also, what are you going to do with the impurities? Do not throw them away or discard them, because they are really delicious, when heated a little and mixed with molasses. Spread all over your toasted bread and eat.

Clarified butter is highly concentrated. That is why it is a bit difficult to digest, when eaten on its own. However, as it is a staple, for giving and nourishing elderly people, it is always mixed up in their vegetables, meat, or beans so that it is easier to digest.

Recognizing Pure Clarified Butter

So how are you going to recognize pure clarified butter, especially when you go to a shop, and ask for butter oil or clarified butter or ghee? Here is the traditional way in which you can find, if the butter has been adulterated with any other oil product or milk products.

Pick up a dried clay pot or utensil and rub some clarified butter on the surface. After a while, if you see a layer of white, where they should be absolutely no layer, that means it has been adulterated.

Take a glass bowl, and add a little bit of mustard oil to it. Now add a little bit of this clarified butter which you bought from the market to it, if there is any adulteration and the clarified butter is not hundred percent pure, it is going to float on the surface of the mustard oil. However, if it is pure, it is going to sink right to the bottom of the glass bowl.

When I told all my friends these two time-tested methods in nodded to take up the purity of clarified butter, they went around making the lives of all the shopkeepers in the vicinity miserable by asking for a test done immediately. And being quite bossy type of voluble ladies, they managed to entertain the whole market, especially when they asked for some of the well-known Agro dairy companies' clarified butter products to be tested then and there.

In fact, one poor beleaguered shopkeeper requested them to go grab hold of those particular companies' top people's throats, instead of shouting at him, he was just the innocent bystander, selling their products! This supposedly very expensive clarified butter is often made up of a mixture of different vegetable oils, to which the essence of clarified butter is mixed and then packaged and sold as hundred percent clarified butter.

In ancient times, people used to purify the air of their houses by taking a piece of dried cow dung, and burning it. On the flames, they added one fourth of a teaspoonful of rice, and one teaspoonful of clarified butter. This gave rise – no pun intended – to lots of smoke, which would have brought out the air pollution authorities to your doorstep, right away or having your smoke alarms clanging clamorously.

Nevertheless, this is the combination of rice and clarified butter, which is burned on cow dung cakes, in traditional Hindu religious ceremonies. Even now, whenever one is having a religious ceremony and wants a "Havan" done, to bless the home or the new born child or anything auspicious the priest is going to burn clarified butter in an altar made up of a fire of sandalwood, if the person is really rich or cow dung cakes if he wants to go in for the really traditional ceremony.

Clarified butter is not good for people suffering from heart problems. However, as it has a resource of vitamin A, they should not stop eating it completely. Instead, they should continue eating it in small amounts in order to keep up with the nutrition. Also, they have to go for walks, and exercise so that the clarified butter is digested properly.

Clarified Butter for Beauty

Remember that clarified butter has a very strong aroma, so if you find any beauty around you smelling of clarified butter, just move away from the vicinity. She has applied it all over her face in order to keep her skin smooth and wrinkle free, free of blemishes, and well moisturized.

I remember as a child going to one of my relatives houses in the ancestral village. Being brought up in the woods and in areas and states away from my native "land", I definitely found the aroma of buttermilk and clarified butter overpowering. Nearly every grand aunt, grand relative, aunt, uncle, and other relative coming to hug us children and telling us how much we had grown smelled overpoweringly of buttermilk and clarified butter.

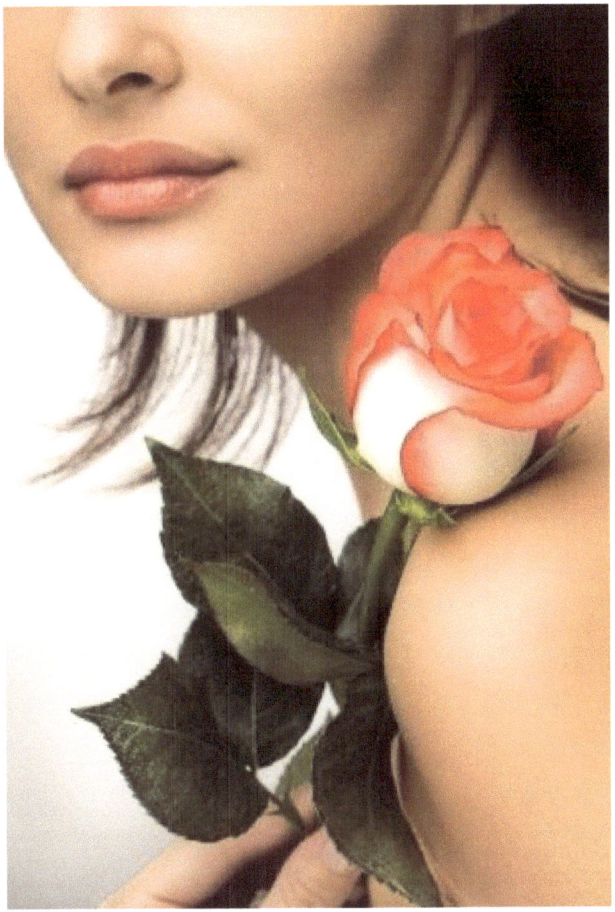

On the plus side, they had beautiful complexions, all soft and well moisturized and wrinkle free, even though some of them were in their 60s. Also, many of them had a very healthy head of hair, shining, soft, and very healthy. This was because every Sunday, they used to rope in one of the idle members of the family to rub their hair, body, and scalps with clarified butter.

Sunday was definitely a day, when we asked our father to take us far far away from the aromatic atmosphere! After that, they basked in the sun like turtles, until it was time for a bath anywhere between 4 to 6 hours later, depending on their moods.

Chronic Migraine

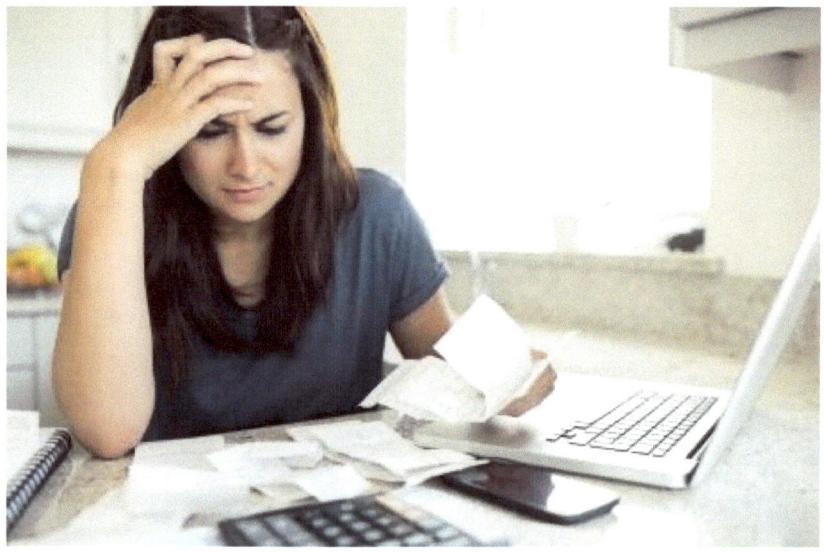

I know of a friend, who woke up with a headache or her sleep got interrupted with an extremely piercing pain in the head. And then she spent the rest of the hours untill waking time wondering which a doctor to meet next the very next morning in order to hunt for a cure.

Then one fine day an Elder told her that her cure was right at hand and very easy. All she had to do was to massage the soles of her feet with clarified butter, every night, before going to sleep. She was cured in four days. I did not believe that until I tried it out for my own headaches.

Apart from the massaging on the soles of the feet as a cure for headaches, I noticed that these headaches occur if there was no oxygen in the room, or if the room was very cold. So you may want to look at these factors also, if you wake up in the middle of the night with your head, aching horribly.

Either close the window or fling open the window.

Laxatives

Try this before you use any sort of laxative. Take a teaspoonful of clarified butter with four peppercorns ground up, every morning for three days. This is going to strengthen your digestive system and make your intestines more receptive to laxatives. On the fourth day, you can use a laxative and this is going to clear out your system. You can also clear out your system by drinking hot milk in which you have added one teaspoonful of clarified butter. This is also an excellent constipation cure.

Wounds and Hurts

This was practiced on me, during one of my jaunts in the hills when I slipped on some rocks, and gashed myself really badly. The moment I reached back home, my host immediately took a piece of cotton and wetted it in water. After that, he wrung it out. This wad of cotton was then placed in a small bowl full of clarified butter and allowed to boil. When all the water content in the cotton wad had evaporated, the ball was taken of the heat, and the cotton wad allowed to cool to lukewarm. All my wounds, 12 of them, small and big were thus bandaged with 12 little warm cotton wads drenched in heated clarified butter.

These were then bandaged. Every morning, the process was repeated and I have absolutely no infection or any scars, remaining of that particular day's activities done on a rainy day in the mountains.

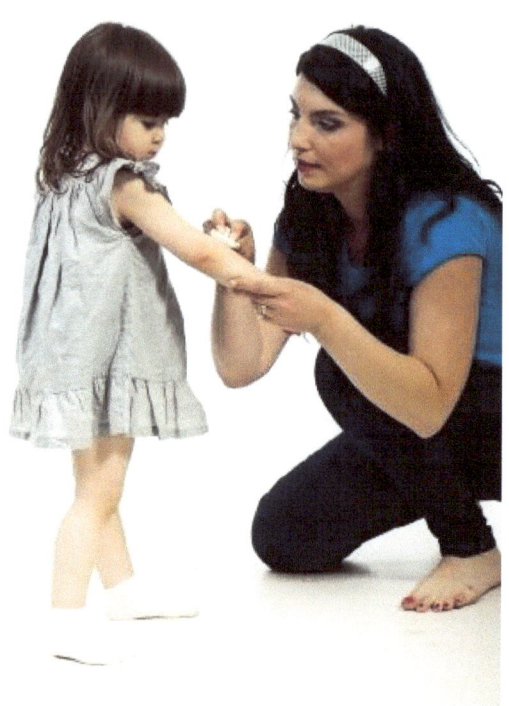

When I asked my host – being a little bit of a tightwad – that he was wasting a whole bowlful of clarified butter in order to prepare a natural herbal cure for me, he just smiled and said that he kept this pure butter for ages by just boiling a betel leaf in it. After that, this was filtered and placed in a glass jar. It remained fresh for ages.

Insomnia

For all those people suffering from insomnia, here is a time-tested remedy. Warm eight drops of clarified butter until they are lukewarm. Now put two – two drops each in your nostrils and inhale. Now put the rest of the four drops in your navel. Now make circular movements in your navel with your finger three anticlockwise and three clockwise.

After that massage the bottom portions of your feet with some warm clarified butter and then drop off to sleep without even bothering about any sort of word called insomnia.

Joint Pain and Gout

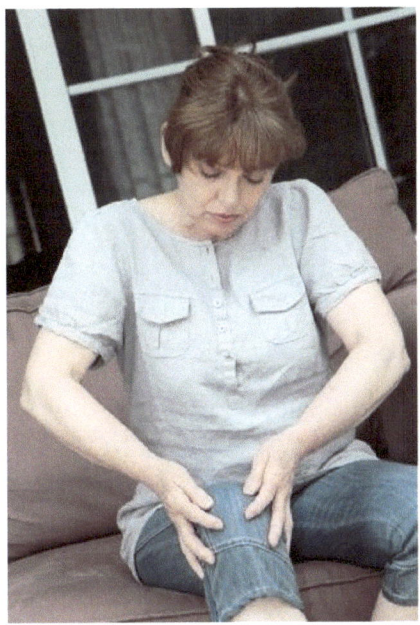

Joint pain is something of which many people suffer especially in the winter. Try massaging the affected area with clarified butter, which has been warmed up. Massage in circular motions all over the affected area. Let me tell you one interesting thing about massaging.

I saw one of these ancient practitioners massaging one of his patients with warm clarified butter. I noticed that he was using three of his fingers – the middle finger, the ring finger and the little finger. The index finger was not being used.

When I asked him why he was using just three fingers, when he could use the full hand to massage his patient, he told me that the index finger – the one with which you point to your antagonist so imperatively or point upwards to make a point, is definitely not beneficial for your health.

Any massage done where you have used the index finger will not show any sort of benefit. He told me that if I was stupid enough to test it out, I could do so. He told me that the next time I cut myself accidentally – so what is new – I should apply the ointment, using the index finger.

The very next morning I cut myself on the rim of an opened cheese tin. So I dipped my index finger into some antiseptic ointment and spread it all over the shallow cut. It took 11 days for that shallow cut to close up and that was only when I stopped using my index finger to apply the ointment.

No wonder some people are so worried about their wounds, not healing properly, that they keep running to the doctor for sugar tests and possibility of diabetes tests.

Cramps

If you are suffering from cramps, which normally occur in hands, feet, thighs, calves, and other parts of your body, note the side of the body which has been cramped. If it occurs in your left side, pull the little finger and the index finger and the little toe and the index toe of your right hand or foot.

And vice versa, if the cramps are on the right side, in which case, you are going to pull your index finger and little finger of your left hand or the index toe and little toe of your left foot.

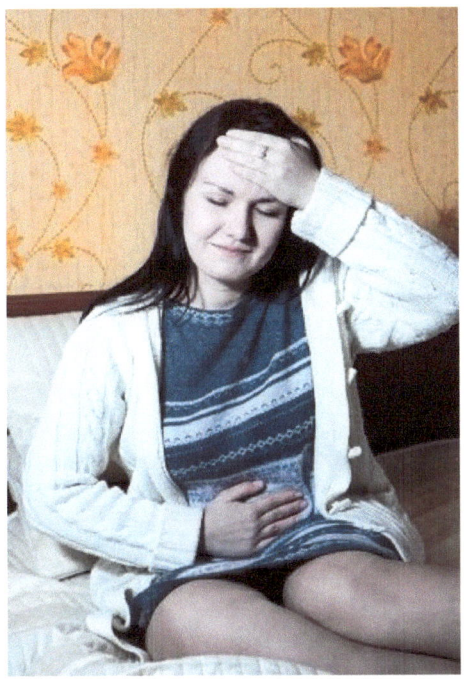

Remember to stretch out your hand or your foot to its fullest extent, when you are doing this. This is an acupuncture trick. This is known to get rid of the cramps immediately.

However, if there is a cramp in your foot then you are going to pull the little finger and index finger or little toe or index toe of that same foot and hand. For cramps in the rest of the body, you do the pulling of the opposite fingers and toes.

Drink a glassful of hot milk and as the area is going to be painful, massage it gently with warm clarified butter.

Burns

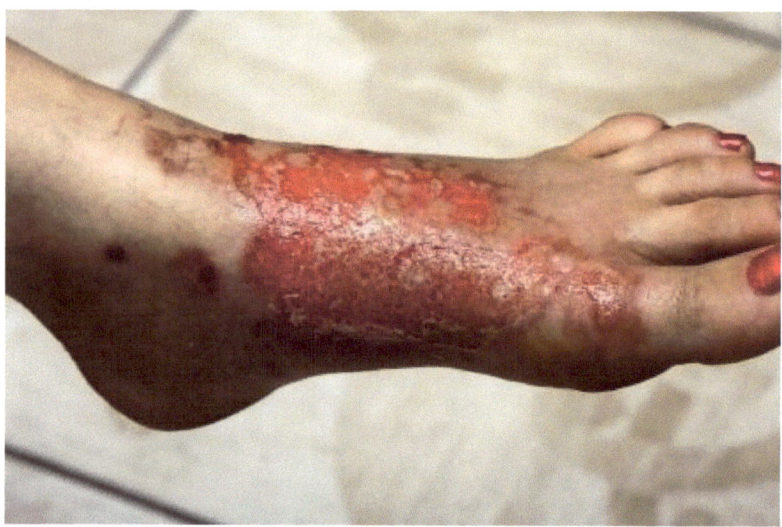

If you have accidentally burned yourself, just apply some warm clarified butter over the affected area. Do not cover or bandage it. This is going to help your burn injuries, without any scars left unless, of course, they are 3rd degree burns, for which you will need to have medical advice and treatment.

Chronic Cough

Take 4 tablespoons full of clarified butter, and add one tablespoonful of molasses to this. Heat the mixture until the molasses are dissolved. Feed the patient this mixture. Along with that, massage the chest area with a mixture of warmed clarified butter in which you have heated a little bit of rock salt. This is excellent for chronic cough.

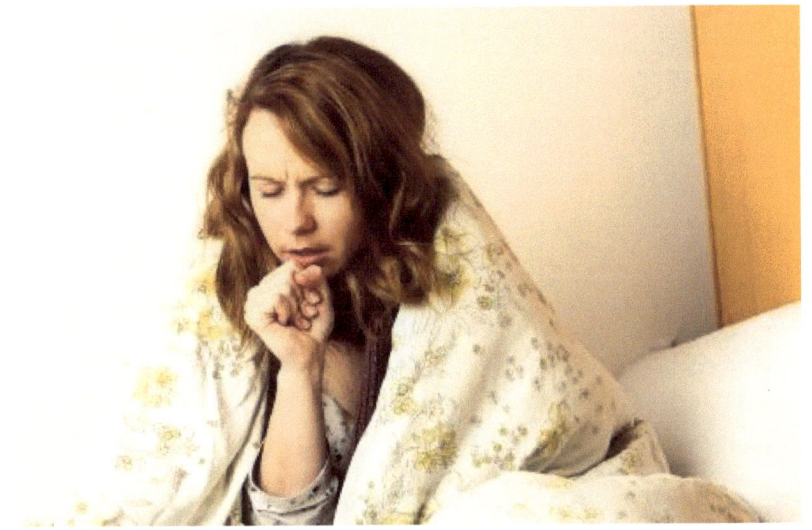

If your cough is winter related take 125 g of milk, and add one tablespoonful of clarified butter to it. Now add 1 cup of water and allow to boil. When this mixture has been reduced to half, add rock candy to it. Drink this four times a day. This is going to get rid of the cough. When we were kids, we demanded this, because this was the only way in which we could drink milk, which it did not taste like milk! Besides, it took care of our cough.

Sore throat

When I was working as a lecturer, I often found myself with a sore throat, because one cannot speak continuously to students for about six hours at a time on different topics without the throat getting affected.

That is why Sunday was a day of total no talking for me! Until one of my public speaker friends told me the best way in which she could make sure that she never suffered from a sore throat due to colds and also a horse throat due to talking on and on and on.

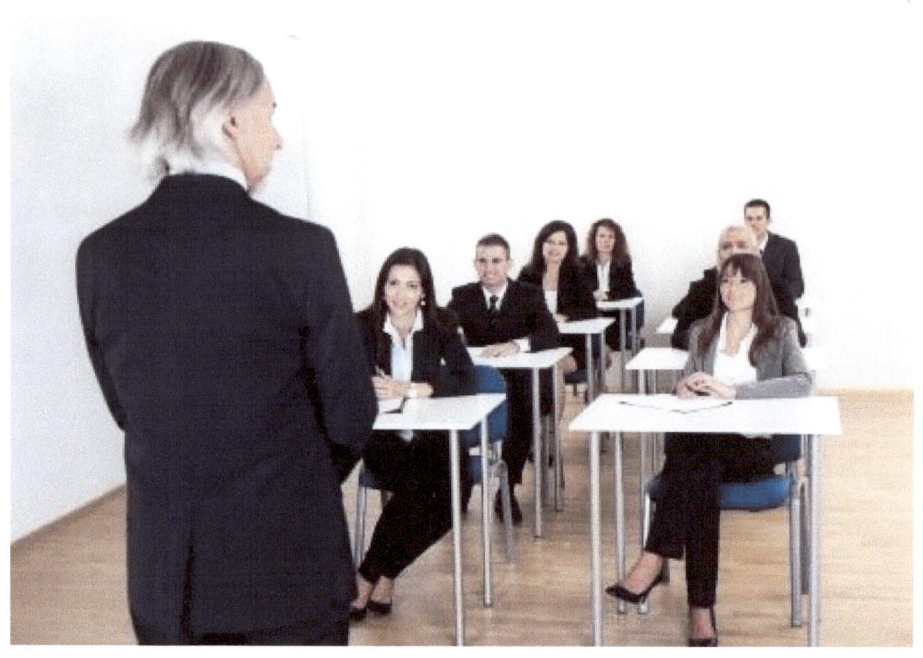

Just take one tablespoonful of clarified butter, one teaspoonful of rock sugar and 15 black peppercorns. Lick the spoon morning and evening. And this is going to get rid of dry cough, a sore throat, and even a hoarse throat. Do not drink any water for a couple of hours after you have taken this remedy. Also, you can take a mixture of warm clarified butter in which you have added some powdered peppercorns, heated it, and allow to cool. This is also excellent for sore throats and that croaking voice.

Colds

If you have a running cold with, especially with watery discharge making you miserable, just take a little bit of clarified butter and warm it. Now dip one finger – not your index finger! – in this warm butter and apply in the inner side of your nostrils. After that, put one drop of this warm clarified butter inside your nostrils and inhale. You are immediately going to find a visible clearing up of your system and ease of breathing.

Do this again after 10 minutes. After that, do it after one hour. And then do that as you wish, because your cold and your running nose have already begun to heal.

Conclusion

This book has given you plenty of time tested and effective remedies for taking care of a number of ailments and diseases. Remember that buttermilk has been called the food of the gods because it helps in curing a large number of these ailments. So if you have not added fresh buttermilk to your diet, you would want to begin drinking it for breakfast and with your lunch.

And if anybody starts whistling "chubby cheeks, dimpled chin, rosy lips, teeth within, curly hair, very fair...", in your vicinity just shrug and blame the buttermilk.

Live Long and Prosper!

Author Bio

Dueep Jyot Singh is a Management and IT Professional who managed to gather Postgraduate qualifications in Management and English and Degrees in Science, French and Education while pursuing different enjoyable career options like being an hospital administrator, IT,SEO and HRD Database Manager/ trainer, movie , radio and TV scriptwriter, theatre artiste and public speaker, lecturer in French, Marketing and Advertising, ex-Editor of Hearts On Fire (now known as Solstice) Books Missouri USA, advice columnist and cartoonist, publisher and Aviation School trainer, ex-moderator on Medico.in, banker, student councilor ,travelogue writer … among other things!

One fine morning, she decided that she had enough of killing herself by Degrees and went back to her first love -- writing. It's more enjoyable! She already has 48 published academic and 14 fiction- in- different- genre books under her belt.

When she is not designing websites or making Graphic design illustrations for clients , she is browsing through old bookshops hunting for treasures, of which she has an enviable collection – including R.L. Stevenson, O.Henry, Dornford Yates, Maurice Walsh, De Maupassant, Victor Hugo, Sapper, C.N. Williamson, "Bartimeus" and the crown of her collection- Dickens "The Old Curiosity Shop," and "Martin Chuzzlewit" and so on… Just call her "Renaissance Woman" - collecting herbal remedies, acting like Universal Helping Hand/Agony Aunt, or escaping to her dear mountains for a bit of exploring, collecting herbs and plants, and trekking.

Check out some of the other JD-Biz Publishing books

Gardening Series on Amazon

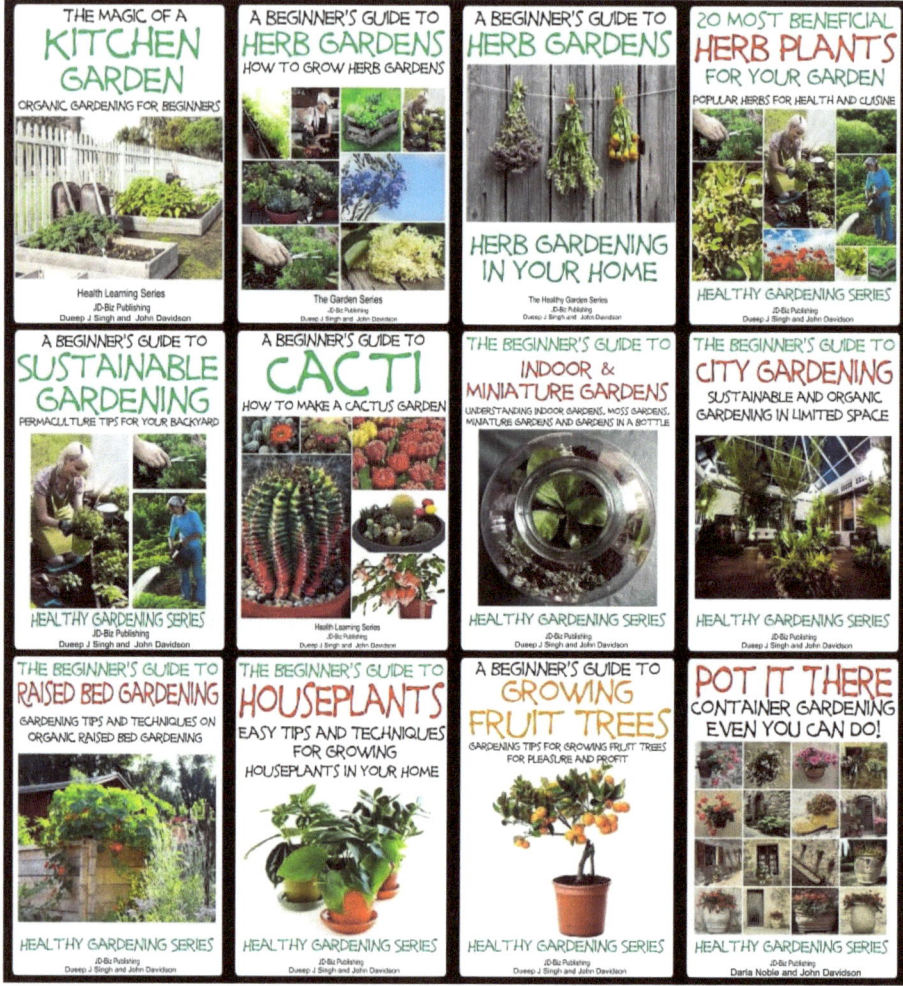

Download Free Books!

http://MendonCottageBooks.com

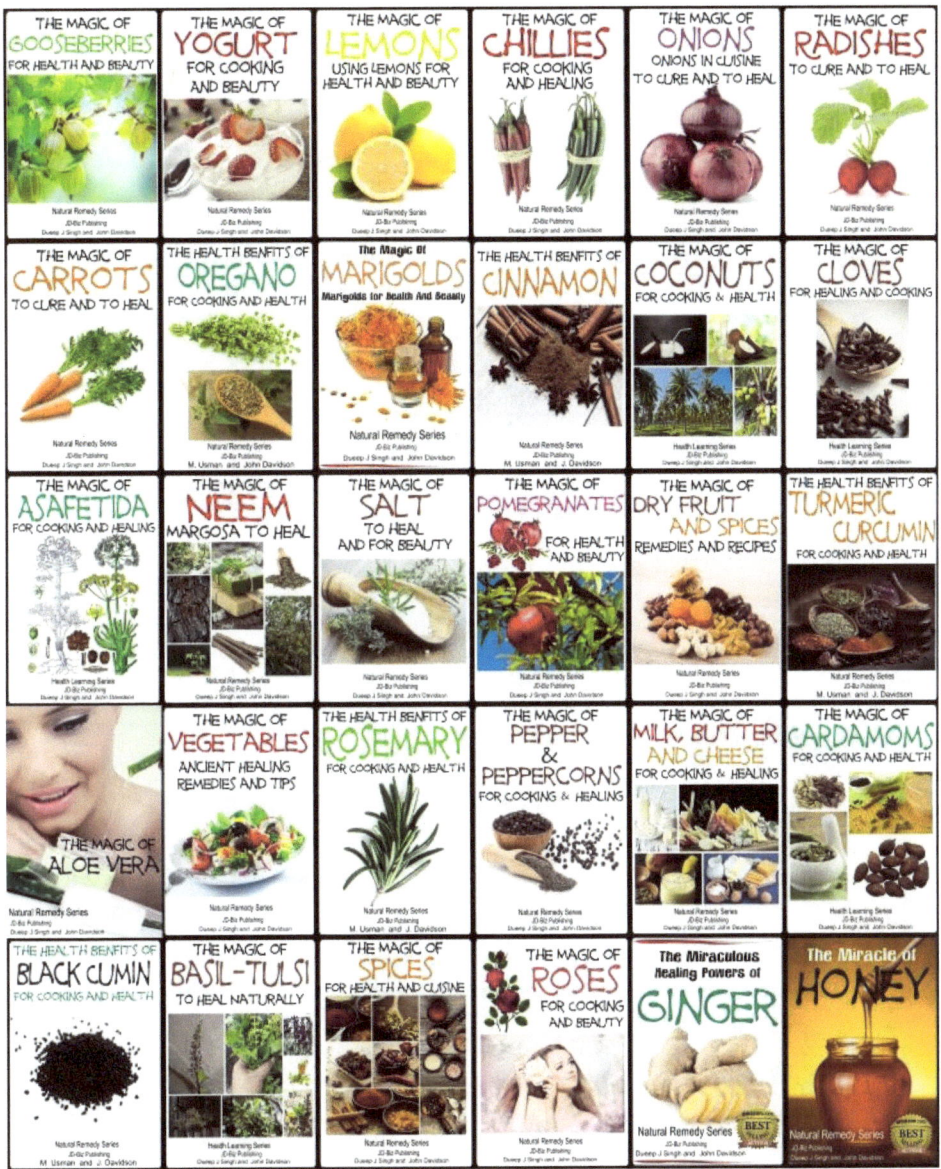

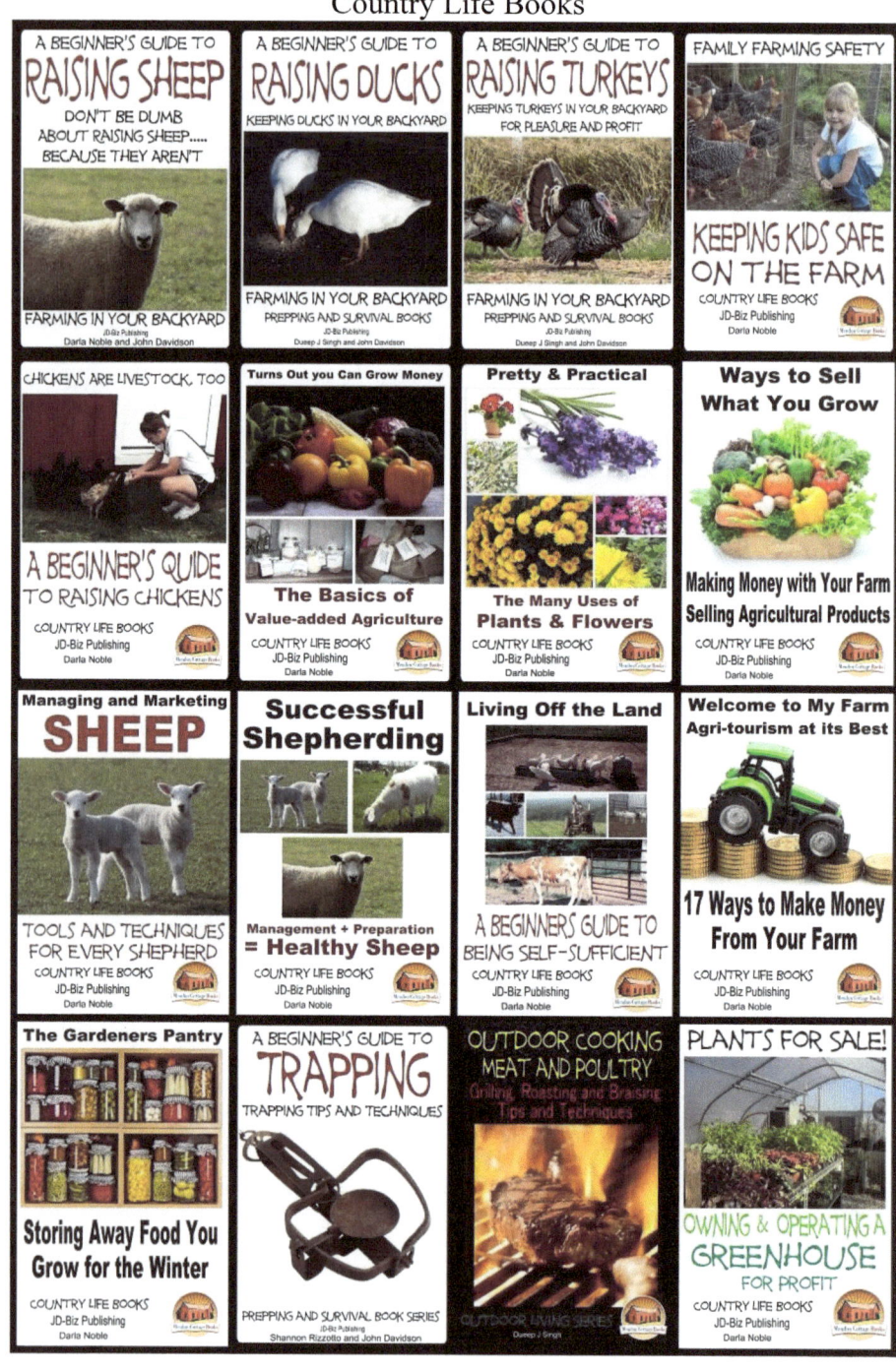

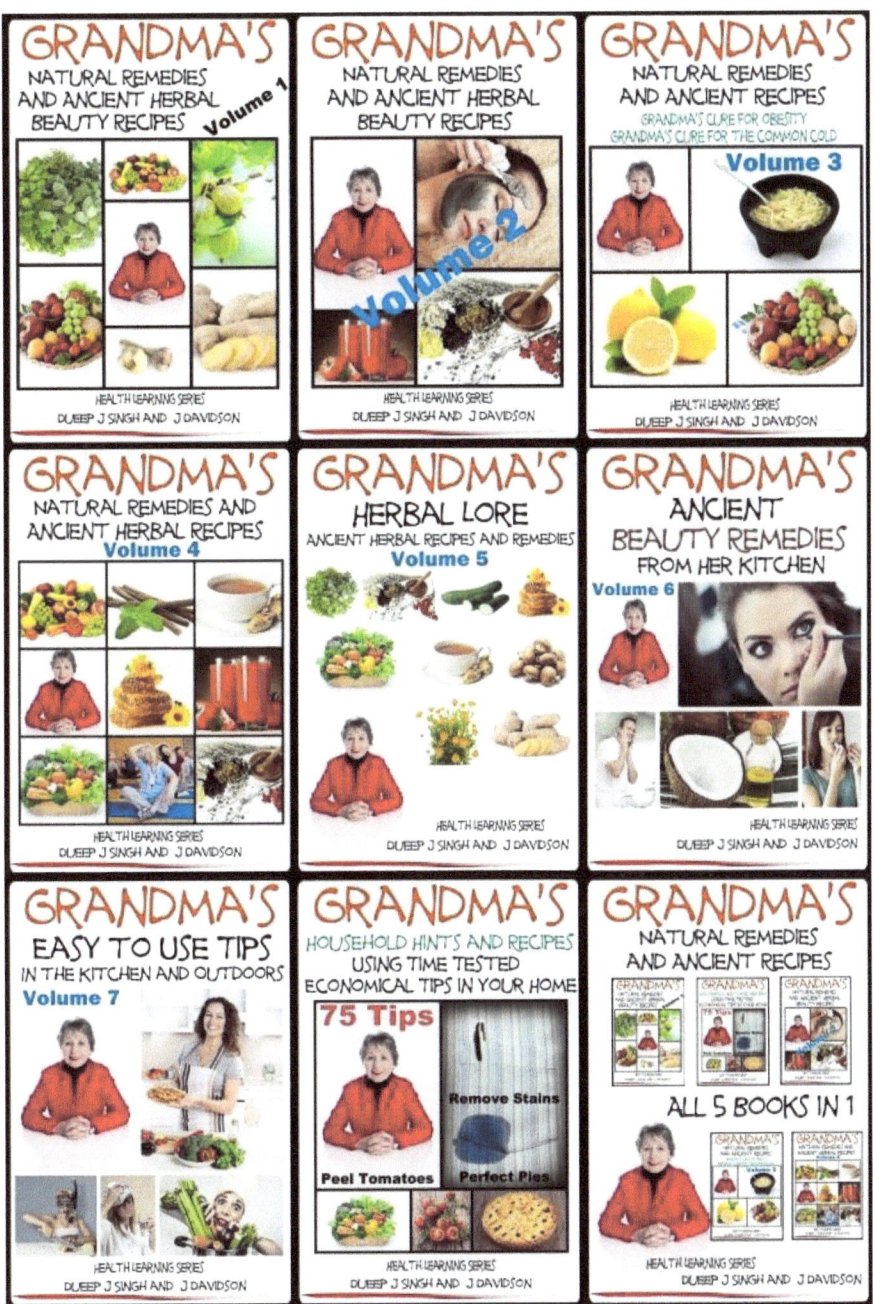

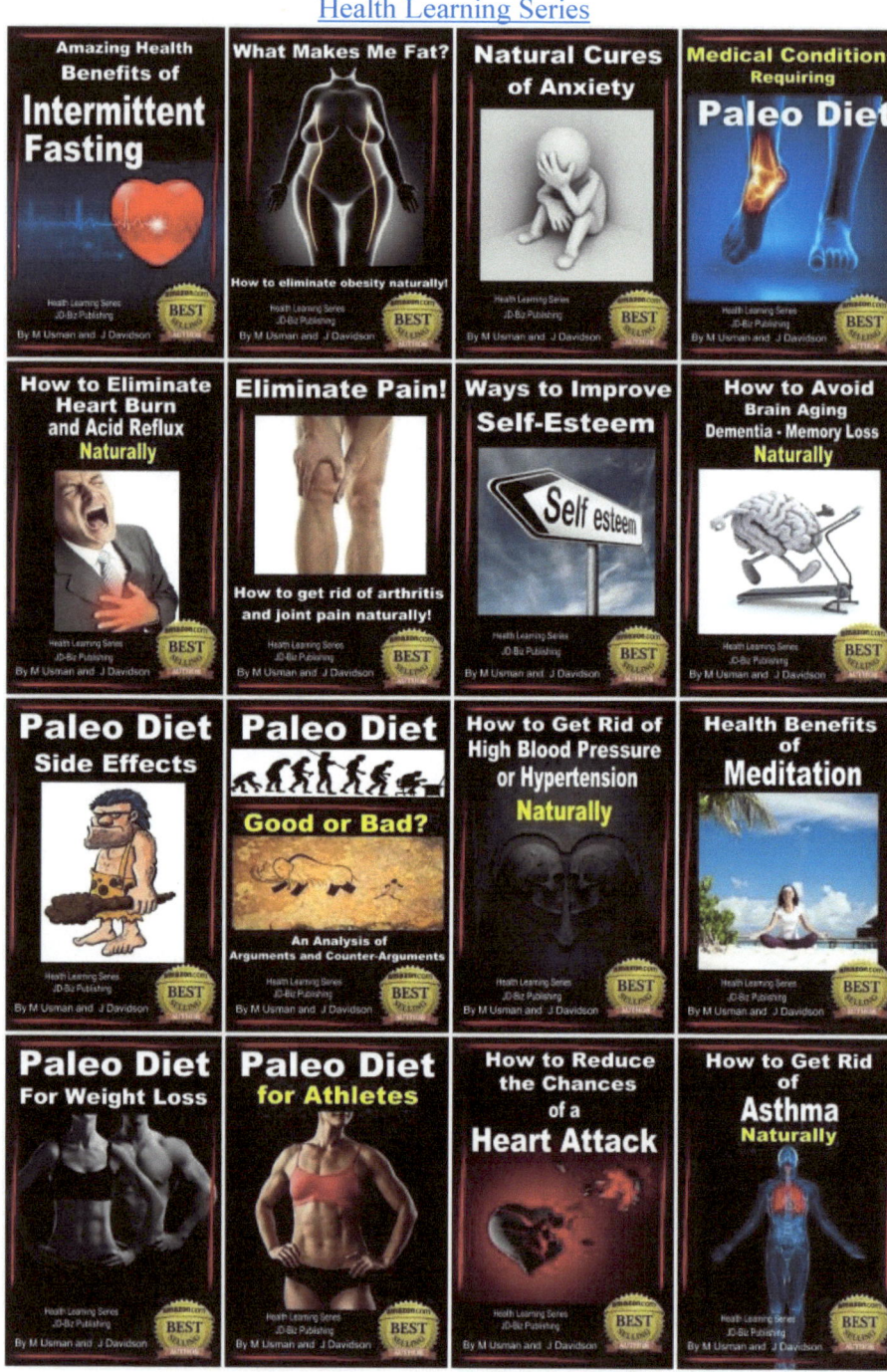

Amazing Animal Book Series

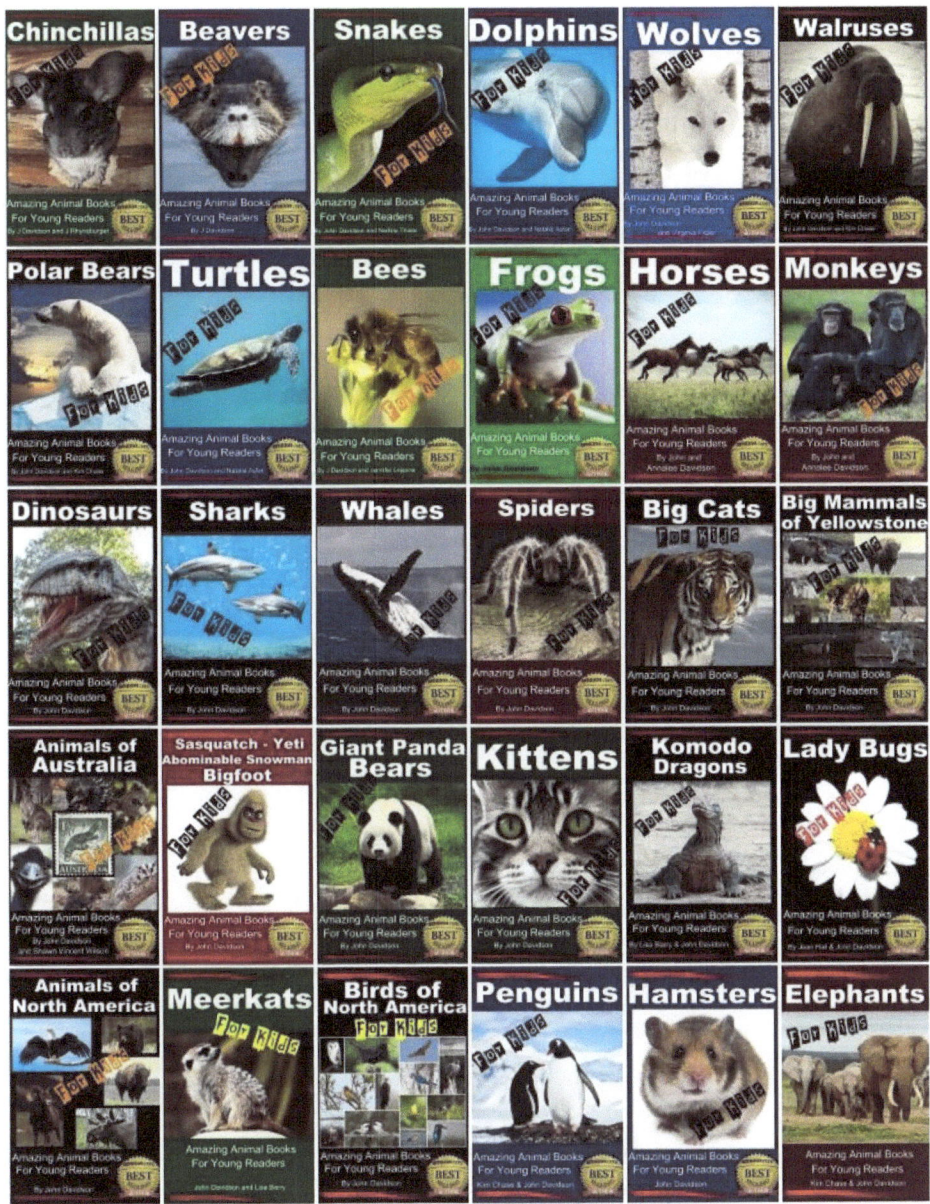

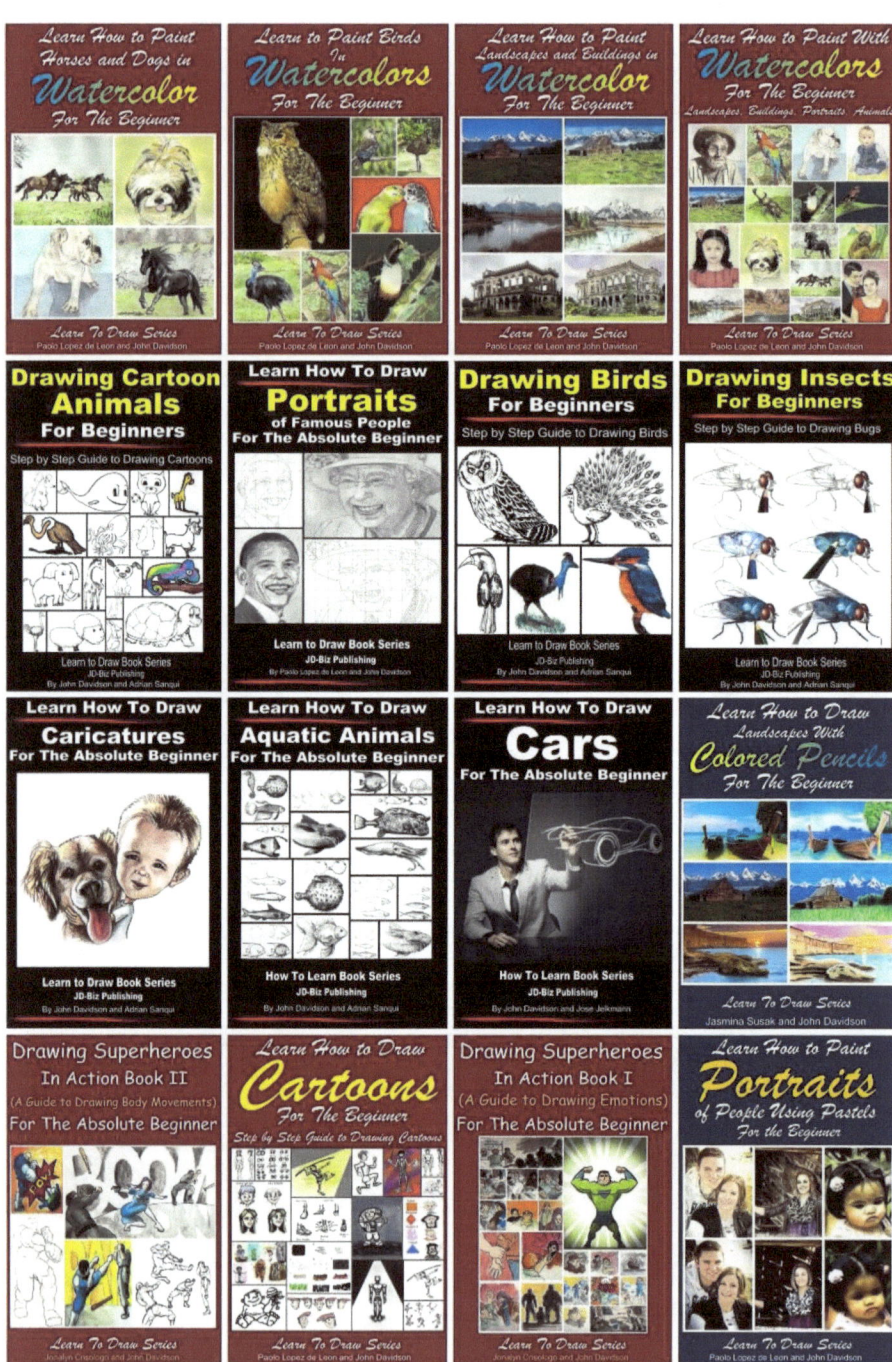

How to Build and Plan Books

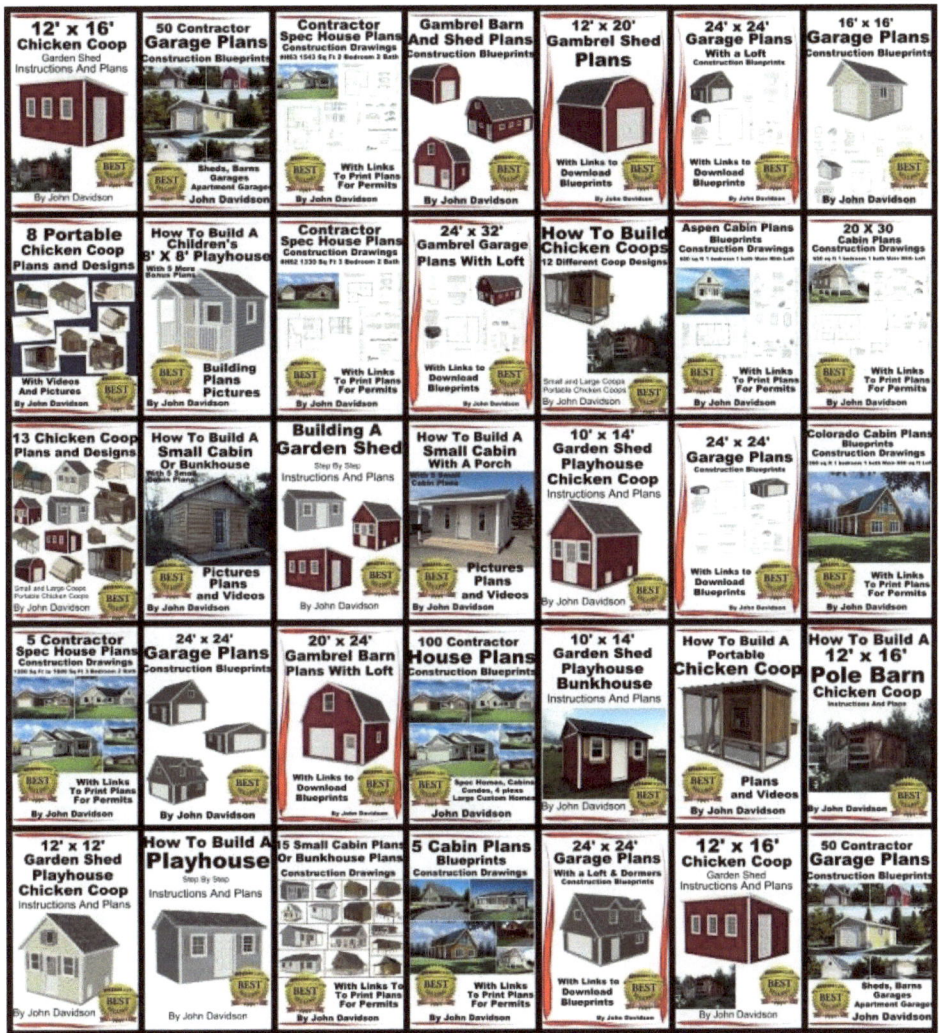

Entrepreneur Book Series

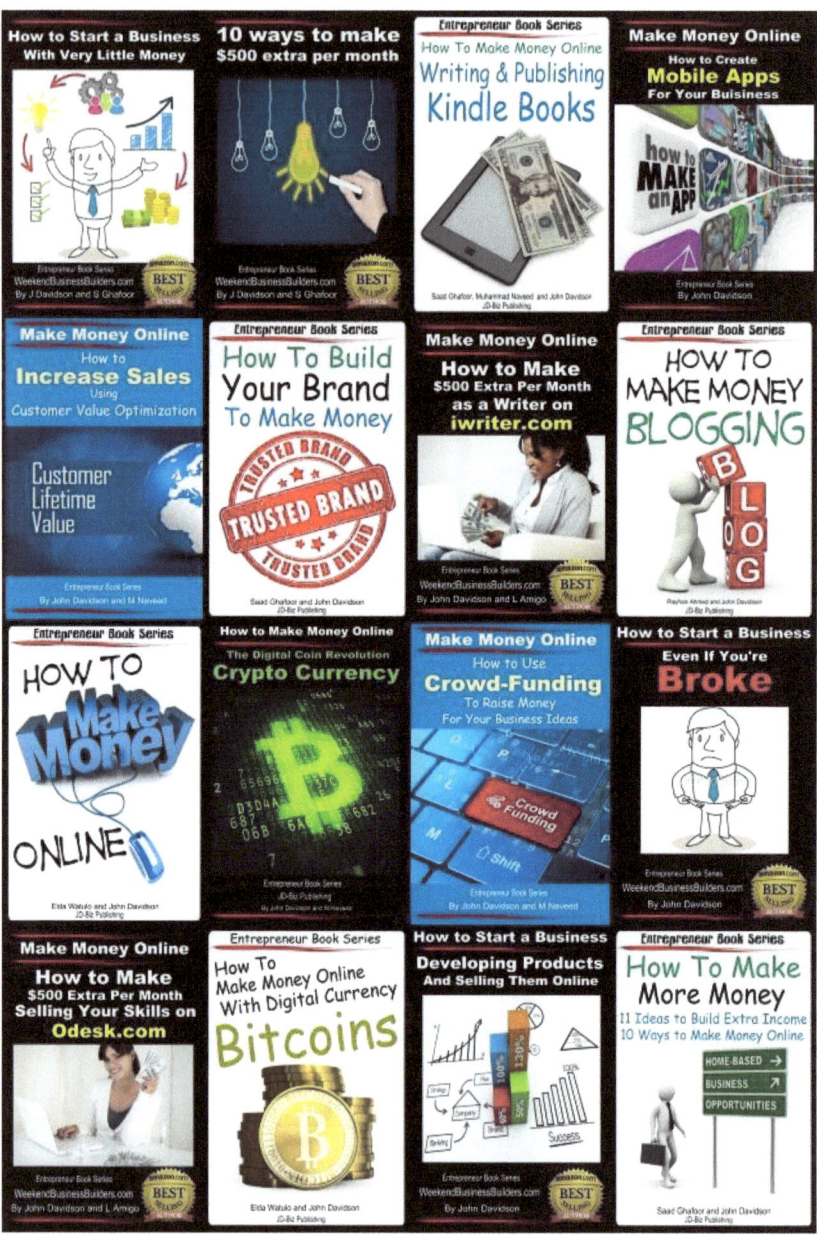

Our books are available at

1. Amazon.com

2. Barnes and Noble

3. Itunes

4. Kobo

5. Smashwords

6. Google Play Books

Download Free Books!

http://MendonCottageBooks.com

Publisher

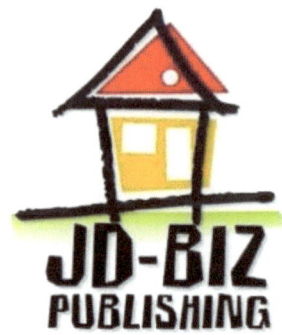

JD-Biz Corp

P O Box 374

Mendon, Utah 84325

http://www.jd-biz.com/

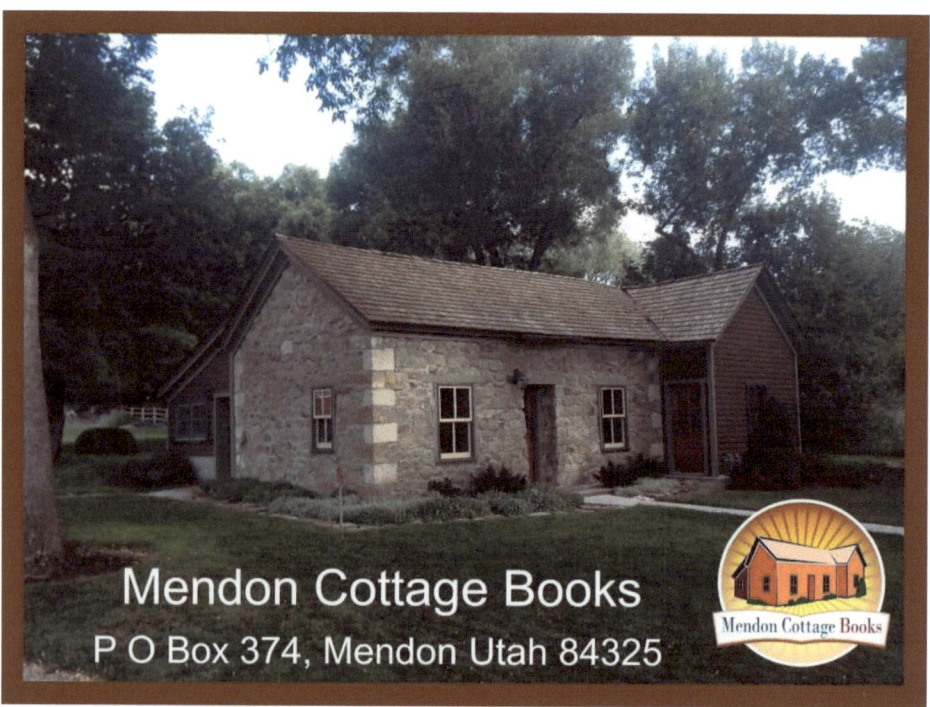

Mendon Cottage Books

P O Box 374, Mendon Utah 84325